A LIFE
OF WELLNESS

Guidelines
For Avoiding Illness

by

Dr. Marty Finkelstein

"A Life of Wellness," by Dr. Marty Finkelstein. ISBN 978-1-60264-204-1.

Copyright 1994 by Dr. Marty Finkelstein. Revised 2008

Manufactured in the United States of America.

Other books and recordings by Dr. Marty Finkelstein

If Relationships were like Sports, Men would at least know the Score
8 Lessons for Life on Hole 1

Moments in Time-CD- 15 original songs

Dedicated To:

My family, friends, and to you and your family and friends who are ready for a "Life of Wellness".

Information>Inspiration>Activation>Transformation

Introduction

I remember walking home from the doctor's office. I was a pre-med student at the University of Oklahoma. I had just received a bachelor's degree in literature. My mother had recently died of ovarian cancer at the early age of fifty-two, and I was searching for answers about life. As I continued to walk, the doctor's words echoed in my heart and head, "You have ulcerative colitis." The medical doctors had explained that this digestive disorder of the large intestine did not have a cure. Simply it was something I would have to learn to live with, and, with the aid of medication, most of the symptoms could be controlled. They explained that if the condition continued to exacerbate, then exploratory surgery would be the next step. I reflected on the last five months of submitting to several diagnostic tests and examinations and taking various drugs to ease abdominal pain. The other host of symptoms I was manifesting was blood in my stool, frequent and irregular bowel movements, difficulty eating and anxiety. All of these symptoms did not add to my social life at the age of twenty-five. I also was told that colitis was a precursor for colon cancer. And, after watching my mom die of cancer, and knowing her brother died of colon cancer at the age of fifty six, it felt as if a dark cloud had been cast over my spirit, even though the sun was shining.

Interestingly, though, when I look back on that day in my life, it probably was the most significant and miraculous in affecting the direction in which I was moving. That day caused me to observe my life differently. Changes I could not foresee were about to take place... physically, emotionally and spiritually. I was about to evolve in ways I could not anticipate.

A few days later, a friend insisted that I see his doctor, a chiropractor. I remember lying on the table, being examined, as the doctor explained about illness and wellness. Instead of learning to live with the problems, he spoke about correcting the cause of the conditions. He shared about holistic wellness and how spiritual, physical, and emotional healing was all integrated. Everything he said made perfect sense. It was while I was lying on his treatment table listening to his words, as well as my own inner conversations, that I had an epiphany and realized what purpose life had for me. I never did take medication after that day, and began to follow the guidelines of healing. If I thought of my illness, as some dark could, I remember it drifting further and further away, as I continued to change my lifestyle, until finally the darkness disappeared. Approximately nine months later I was no longer experiencing pain, and the multitude of symptoms I had. Ulcerative colitis no longer was affecting my body. It was gone! That was over thirty years ago and I have continued to follow the "Life of Wellness" guidelines as I assist others to discover the optimum possibilities for their health.

This book is written so that all of us can begin the process of wellness before crisis occurs as well as recognizing what we can do when a disease process has already begun. There are excellent books that cover this information in depth, but this book is a simple map that outlines the journey and keeps the destination clearly in focus.

As doctors, we can assist our patients the most when they are involved in the responsibility and understanding of their own health.

This is a book that can be read again and again. It can also be given to children so that they can begin knowing their inner voice never needs to be lost, and that "A Life of Wellness" should be anticipated.

—Beginning—

It was his time to be born soon. In the peaceful dark space of the womb the voices shared with him many stories about the transitions of Living.

They had also told him how much is forgotten once born about health, healing, and the true nature of who we are. Sadly he knew he was coming into a world where illness and disease were accepted as a normal occurrence of life and how people used drugs routinely to numb physical and emotional pains.

The voices told him that more faith had been placed in medicine and surgery than in the natural healing powers of the Divine Intelligence that had created everything and everyone.

If people could only see what I see, he thought. He breathed deeply and gazed at all the miracles before him. The voices shared with him that everything was designed by the Creator. That his body and mind, feelings and thoughts were meant to function in harmony, guided by a healing wisdom that always could be listened to and observed.

But the voices told him how easy it was for people to lose their natural understanding of nurturing and caring for their body and mind.

Even as he prepared for his own birth the voices told how the birthing process itself had become a time of trauma, interfered by medication and sometimes surgery. He learned that many if not all the stories he had heard during his development would be forgotten. The magic, the miracles, the wisdom, the voices, the Creator, all would disappear as the numbing of drugs and more drugs became a lifestyle. He sighed as he observed the wonderful workings of his mind and body. What a marvelous thing a human being is, he thought. He knew he was a part of the Creator, and yet what a wonderful gift the Creator had given him.

He was aware of his beingness.....

Seeing, hearing, smelling, feeling, tasting, and knowing. How would people take care of themselves differently if they never stopped knowing, he wondered?

What if they could reawaken to what was so obvious from inside here? He already knew all things were possible. It was just a matter of everyone remembering and knowing again.

He knew his time was coming. He knew a new lifetime was about to begin. In his last thoughts before being born, he prayed that he would remember.

That he would remember the stores the magic, the miracles, the voices, and the Creator.

−1−

You were divinely created in approximately nine months by an Innate Wisdom that knows exactly what to do.

From the merging of two microscopic cells you came into life.

Hopefully your birth was without drugs and surgical interventions.

–2–

Your life is about learning how to take care of this marvelous gift. By maximizing your unique potential you can unfold to the many blessings of life.

When the time comes it is about sharing this wisdom with the children of the world.

–3–

When you speak of the mind and body you speak of it as separate parts of you.

But the mindbody works simultaneously together. There is nothing that is just in your mind or just in your body.

You are a mindbody.

Every thought and feeling influence
Our mindbody.

–4–

Physical sensations affect you emotionally, and emotional feelings affect you physically. There is always a direct connection to your mindbody's wholeness.

Observe your mindbody when you feel anger, joy, fear, love, depression, and excitement.

−5−

When you begin to observe how your mindbody works together, you will have taken the first steps toward your own responsibility and the potential health and wellness in your life.

–6–

Your beliefs regarding your health will directly influence the actions you take.

Your beliefs are not necessarily thoughts or ideas that you have voted on or contemplated.

Your beliefs may not be true.

After all, the earth is not flat… or is it?

−7−

Information, education, and experience, or the lack of these, will shape your beliefs.

If your beliefs seem to limit your potential either physically, emotionally, or spiritually, then consider why you have those beliefs and where they came from.

–8–

The steps that you take to become healthier are:

Changing the beliefs that rob you of your own potential wellness,

and developing a new attitude that seeks out improvement in your lifestyle.

–9–

If you believe nothing can be done for

    Your health problems

    You will do nothing.

If you believe your problems exist simply

    Because you are getting older,

    You will do nothing.

If you believe it is just stress,

    You will do nothing….

And the problems will continue to get worse.

–10–

Imagine your mindbody like the most sophisticated computer in which you have only used five percent of its potential.

Imagine now having access into the other ninety-five percent which you did not know existed.

–11–

The good news is that there are genetic and hereditary influences regarding your health that you cannot change or control… so don't worry about those.

But the greatest news is that there are many factors regarding your health that you can change and influence.

That is what this book is about.

–12–

There has been an increase of illness in our society, an increase of surgery, and an increase of medication. The focus of health care has been toward crisis intervention rather than wellness and optimal health.

–13–

If more time was spent educating adults and children about wellness and healthy lifestyles, not only would you benefit and reap the rewards…

But health care costs would also be tremendously diminished in the process.

–14–

Most illnesses in our society could be prevented by a total commitment toward creating healthy lifestyles and by understanding that the more you learn to take care of yourself, the more productive you become in living your life.

–15–

Becoming healthier and enjoying the benefits of a healthy lifestyle is more than just crossing fingers and hoping.

You have to be involved in the process of your own potential wellness.

–16–

Whether you call it God, Creator, Power, Innate Wisdom, Nature, or Life itself, that essence does *its* part and you are here to do *your* part.

Imagine God has given you the gift of life.

Imagine your gift back to God is to nurture this life.

–17–

The symptoms in your body were never meant to be masked, numbed, ignored, or adapted to.

Symptoms are the way the mindbody's wisdom gets your attention. Behind every symptom is a cause. Behind every cause is an opportunity of improving your overall health.

–18–

The decisions you choose when you experience any symptom determine which direction you are moving toward.

Symptoms occur to guide you and teach you something about yourself.

–19–

Headaches, anxiety, indigestion, back pains, cramps, stress, fatigue, allergies, depression, fear, anger, stiffness, and shortness of breath are all symptoms.

–20–

If a symptom is treated without treating the cause of the problem it will continue to get worse and eventually cause other complicated symptoms. Throughout this process your mindbody's resistance weakens to the inevitable manifestation of further illness.

–21–

Cancer, heart disease, arthritis, diabetes, osteoporosis, and strokes all take years to develop, and are the manifestations of the mindbody's defenses being weakened.

Once these diseases are diagnosed, they continue in their own process of degeneration, unless the causes of these conditions are treated.

–22–

All medications have side effects and adverse reactions. The optimal goal is to never need medication. If taking medication is necessary, as it might be for crisis intervention, discover what wellness steps can be taken to reduce that necessity. Without increasing the wellness factor, the mindbody continues to adapt and lead to further illnesses.

–23–

Always ask your medical doctor what can be done besides medication or in addition to medication. The goal is to strengthen your health and assist your immune system and nervous system in functioning at their maximum healing capacity.

–24–

Most of us have been raised on a crisis model of health rather than on a wellness model. Medication has been the standard of treatment since birth itself.

More and more babies are raised on medication, starting with allergies, ear infections, colic, colds, fevers, and asthma. Sadly, the cycle continues as the child gets older. Medication becomes a lifestyle, as illness and symptoms are regarded as a normal response to life.

–25–

Using medicine for symptoms without finding out what is causing the dysfunction is like taking a pain pill for a toothache and not consulting a dentist to find what is causing the pain.

At one time people thought it was normal to lose our teeth by the time we were forty years old. The only time people went to the dentist was to have their teeth pulled out. What health problems do you have that you think are normal?

–26–

Drugs and medicine have a specific purpose in reducing symptoms and assisting the mindbody in a crisis. Drugs and medicine were never meant to be a lifestyle. Drugs and medicine do not assist you in becoming healthier.

–27–

Your mind body can adapt and compensate to most problems you have. The more chronic your problem becomes, the higher your pain threshold becomes.

Your goal should not be to determine what you can get used to, or live with, but to strengthen and enhance the mindbody's healing power.

–28–

Your mind body can get used to just about everything. Regardless of how complicated your problems are, it is easy to think, "It's not that bad".

The question is, why would you want to adapt to a problem if you don't have to?

–29–

Always know the side effects and contraindications of every medication you take.

If medicine and drugs actually helped us to become healthier, we should be the healthiest people alive.

–30–

Your immune system is your defense system. The continuous lifestyle of medication from aspirin to antibiotics, from allergy pills to digestive tablets, weakens the process of how all the systems in our mindbody are designed to function.

–31–

It is easy to understand why taking medication is part of most lifestyles.

1. It is easy.
2. It offers quick relief of symptoms.
3. It does not require a change in your lifestyle.
4. It is a habit. You have been taking medications since childhood.
5. Our society continues to promote medicine as a symptom and prevention choice.

–32–

Taking medicine can sometimes add years to your life, but learning about your health and becoming an active participant in your health will add life to your years.

−33−

Just imagine not taking medication for every symptom you have; instead, listening to why your mindbody is attempting to get your attention.

Allow the wisdom of your mindbody to be heard.

Imagine you were listening to your mindbody as if it were brand new Cadillac rather than a fifty-four Chevy. How would you treat it differently?

–34–

Wellness is a process like illness. If you want further wellness, you have to be involved with the steps of manifesting this in your life. The benefits are:

1. More energy
2. More flexibility
3. More creativity
4. More concentration and focus in your life
5. More expression of joy and love
6. More strength and endurance
7. A better relationship with friends and family
8. Aging with grace and vitality
9. Intimate passionate relationships
10. A deeper spiritual understanding of life

–35–

Wellness is no different from anything else in your life. Those areas in your life where you have achieved success are areas in your life where you have devoted time and commitment.

So how devoted have you been toward taking care of yourself?

–36–

As your wellness becomes a top priority, everything else in your life will improve as well.

The more time you spend to take care of yourself the more time you will have to take care of everything else.

–37–

You live in a fast-paced world. No one has more than twenty-fours in the day. You must make the time to take care of your health and optimum wellness. The more it seems that you don't have the time, the more important it becomes to reevaluate your lifestyle.

Don't wait for a crisis to get your attention.

–38–

Most people are familiar with yearly medical examinations to evaluate illness and disease, yet these examinations do not evaluate how healthy you are.

–39–

When your medical doctor says you checked out fine, but prescribes some medication for your indigestion, he means he did not find any tumors, broken bones, improper blood chemistry, or diagnosed diseases.

That is wonderful news, yet something is causing the indigestion.

–40–

Typical Scenario

FIRST EXAM:
Doctor: The results were negative but here is medication for your indigestion.

SECOND EXAM, ONE YEAR LATER:
Doctor: The test results were negative. This new medication is a little stronger for your digestive pain and bloating.

THIRD EXAM, ONE YEAR LATER:

Doctor: The results were negative. This is a new type of medication for the pressure and discomfort.

FOURTH EXAM, ONE YEAR LATER:

Doctor: We found what is causing the problem. There is tumor in your large intestine. It is recommended that we perform exploratory surgery at this time and then follow up with further evaluations.

The patient is happy because he knew all along there was a specific problem. However, he never knew the alternatives in discovering the cause of the symptoms and correcting it before it became more complicated.

What would you do now if you could prevent that tumor from occurring?

Here are good questions to ask doctors:

1. But what is causing my discomfort?
2. What is the medication for?
3. What are the side effects of the medication?
4. Is there anything I can do now to help my problem other than medicine?
5. What illness or disease can these symptoms lead to if the problem continues?

–41–

Sometimes surgery is necessary. Most of the time it is not. Become aware of your alternatives before submitting to surgery. There are wonderful books from specialists in all the various health fields that address alternatives and approaches toward wellness. Begin reading new information about these aspects of your life.

–42–

All the organs in your mind body are there for specific reasons. Learn how to nurture your wellness and keep your organs for your entire life.

–43–

Illness and wellness are a process rather than a thing. Either you are serving your illness or serving your health.

Everything in your mindbody is constantly changing. Problems get worse when you do not take the proper actions. The mindbody has the best possibilities of healing when you take the proper steps of wellness.

The mind body consists of many systems functioning simultaneously:

1. Digestive System
2. Circulatory System
3. Respiratory System
4. Reproductive System
5. Endocrine System
6. Urinary System
7. Immune System
8. Musculo-Skeletal System
9. Special senses: hearing, tasting, seeing, smelling, feeling

ALL these systems are coordinated and influenced by the Nervous System.

–45–

We all have been raised on medical doctors and medicine.

If you have not yet been to a Chiropractic Doctor, find one.

Chiropractic is the largest natural health profession in the world.

–46–

Chiropractic began in 1895 as a science, an art, and a philosophy. The profession has grown continuously with the understanding that healing comes from within our mindbody. If we reduce the interference to the nervous system then the mindbody can do what it was intended to do. Be healthy, stay healthy, and continue to improve in ALL the possibilities of your potential.

–47–

Chiropractors spend a great amount of time evaluating the cranium, sacrum and the spine and its relationship with the nervous system. The spine protects the spinal cord, where nerves relay messages to every muscle and organ in your body.

–48–

The best way to understand chiropractic treatment and care is by talking with a chiropractor.

Going to a chiropractor does not take the place of going to a medical doctor.

Nor does going to a medical doctor take the place of going to a chiropractor.

–49–

Imagine a medical doctor referring you to a chiropractor before recommending you for surgery or intensive medication.

Imagine your Doctor of chiropractic discussing your health and prognosis with your medical doctor and both committed toward your overall wellness and care.

–50–

Since 1895, chiropractors have assisted people to greater wellness in their lives.

Asthma and allergies in children, arthritis and high blood pressure in adults, headaches and back pain that so many people suffer from, have all been helped through the natural and painless approach of chiropractic treatment.

–51–

Chiropractic treatment is essential in assisting the mindbody's function toward its maximum wellness, regardless of the problems people have.

The wisdom that made this mindbody can heal it, when you learn how to take care of it properly.

–52–

Most of us have been trained and educated to go to medical doctors when we are sick or in pain.

Dentists have educated us how to prevent problems from ever occurring simply by having our teeth examined from early childhood.

–53–

What has worked as a wellness model for our teeth is the same wellness model we should use for the rest of our mindbody.

A lifestyle of wellness begins by having children understand their health by evaluating the developing structure and functioning of the spine and nervous system.

–54–

No one healing profession has all the answers and expertise.

If medical doctors and chiropractors worked toward the same purpose of helping people stay healthy, we would have less illnesses, and less necessity of medication and surgery.

–55–

These are some other natural healing methods that understand the principles of wellness.

1. Acupuncture
2. Naturopathy
3. Homeopathy
4. Ayurvedic
5. Massage
6. Counseling/Psycho-therapy
7. Hypnotherapy
8. Feldenkrais
9. Alexander
10. Reiki
11. Yoga
12. Nutrition

When we integrate many holistic approaches of healing to our health, our life expands. Expanding means that we are having healthier relationships with other people as well as having a healthier relationship with ourselves.

–56–

People do not look forward to getting sick. Sometimes we just don't use our insight and foresight in avoiding sickness.

Compassionately learn from other people's illnesses. It is a good idea to visit a hospital and observe the patients there.

Confirm for yourself that this is not where you want to be. The best way to assist others who are ill is to increase your own wellness.

–57–

No doctor does the healing. Healing occurs from within your mindbody's wisdom. The potential of this power needs to be realized again.

Cancer, Aids, Multiple Sclerosis, and other illness and dysfunctions can be understood as a process that can be reversed, assisted and healed through utilizing the expertise in all healing sciences and arts.

–58–

Healing takes time even when the proper procedures are applied. Broken bones in casts, and braces on teeth need specific time for the potential correction.

Chronic discomfort pain and illnesses need time to heal even when the correct procedures are used.

When the proper procedures are not utilized, the mindbody's communication for optimal healing cannot take place.

–59–

Compensation and adaptation is the mind-body's response when optimum healing is interfered with. Teeth continue to get crooked, broken bones do not mend properly, aggravated muscles continue to get tighter, blood pressure continues to get higher as the heart works harder, and the posture of the physical body seeks out new ways of bending, sitting, and standing to avoid discomfort.

Disease is the byproduct of compensation and adaptation.

–60–

Chiropractors evaluate the spine to determine if there are minor misalignments of the vertebra of the spine. This is called a subluxation complex. Subluxations cause pressure on the nerves that communicate through the spinal pathways from the brain to the rest of the body.

–61–

Subluxations can occur from problems in the womb, at birth, during childhood development, from poor posture, lack of exercise, all types of injuries, improper nutrition, and from physical and emotional stresses.

–62–

Subluxations cause various symptoms for different people. Pressures on the nerves affect the functioning of all parts of your mindbody.

You can have a subluxation, similar to having a cavity and not be aware of it; simply because you are not manifesting symptoms at the time.

–63–

Chiropractors are specialists in reducing, stabilizing, and correcting subluxations, and nerve interference.

Because subluxations can occur from the birth process itself, it is important for babies to be checked by a chiropractor.

–64–

The birth process is a miraculous and wonderful experience.

It is important that the least intervention and interference occur. Natural childbirth without drugs and surgery and surrounded by loved ones, is ideal.

–65–

Remember that every drug that you take during labor, your baby is taking also.

Most Caesarian births are the byproduct of interfering with the natural process of labor and delivery.

–66–

If you have your baby in the hospital, let your doctors know you would like to have a natural childbirth, without drugs.

If you have your childbirth in a hospital, make sure it has a birthing room separate from the rest of the hospital.

–67–

Since health for a new child begins in the womb, make certain you are applying the steps of wellness for yourself and your baby during pregnancy.

–68–

There is no good substitute for mother's milk. Information shows that:

1. Nature knows what it is doing.
2. A bonding between mother and child physically and emotionally continues.
3. The nutrition of mother's milk is perfect for the newborn. The baby's neuro-immune system is strengthened through mother's milk.
4. Bottle-fed babies are usually held on the same side of the body, while breast-fed babies are switched side-to-side allowing both eyes to develop and perceive the outside world.

Bottle-fed babies have more allergies and asthma than breast-fed babies. Babies are then placed on medications with no end in sight. This continues to weaken the immune system making us more susceptible to other problems and continued allergies and asthma.

–70–

Your immune system protects and defends your mindbody. More and more is being discovered how the nervous system and immune system interact together, influencing your illness or your wellness.

Natural immunity can occur by strengthening the neuro-immunal responses by increasing the capacity of your overall wellness.

Every pediatrician should find a chiropractor who would be happy to explain how chiropractic treatment can assist in reducing unnecessary medication for allergies, colds, and asthma.

To often when these conditions are not corrected learning disabilities can occur in young ages. It is necessary for parents to understand natural alternatives for attention deficit disorders.

–72–

Most problems that occur to the mindbody are waiting to happen. Have you ever known someone to say that they were fine, and then the next day couldn't move their back? How about the person who had a heart attack?

Feeling fine does not mean that you are healthy!

–73–

We all have good days and not-so-good days within the rhythms of our lifestyles.

Someone's good day could be a terrible day for you.

The question to ask yourself is, "Am I in the process of improving my health."

–74–

Feeling healthy, being healthy, and becoming healthier can be worlds apart

Chiropractors evaluate the subtleties of your health, assisting you in becoming your best.

Chiropractors observe specific relationships existing between the physical and emotional body that remain unnoticed by other doctors.

–75–

Doctors must serve and educate their patients. If a doctor does not take the time to answer your questions, find another one.

Make certain you take the time to ask questions.

–76–

Before going to a doctor, write down questions you want to be answered.

Also write down any concerns you have about your health.

It is easy to forget these important issues once you are in an office.

–77–

When a doctor says:

It's just your nerves,
It's just stress,
You are just getting older
It's just growing pains,
There is nothing that can be down,
You will just have to learn to live with
it…..

Find another doctor!

–78–

Your health deserves not "just" but

- Justice
- Compassion
- Understanding
- Information
- Possibilities
- Alternatives
- Truth

–79–

When a doctor does not know what your problem is after his evaluations, and examinations, he should say so.

The doctor should talk to you about alternatives.

–80–

Unless the doctor's name is "God," it should never be said that

"Nothing can be done except more drugs and surgery"

or

"You'll just have to learn to live with it.

–81–

There is always something that can be done and should be done. How much can be done and how much healing can take place is the unknown. There are never limitations to the wisdom that created your mindbody.

–82–

Your physical health PLUS
Your emotional health PLUS
Your spiritual health
EQUALS
Your total wellness

They are not separate from each other, but together are a manifestation of who you are.

–83–

Ask your doctor what he or she does to be healthy and stay healthy.

A doctor should be involved in the same process of wellness that he hopes to assist you in.

–84–

Ask your medical doctor to explain surgical procedures if surgery is necessary.

Ask what complications can occur, and what will be necessary after surgery.

Ask what alternatives exist.

–85–

Ask your chiropractic doctor to explain chiropractic treatment and what can be anticipated. Discover the differences between relief care, corrective care, and wellness care.

–86–

Illness in our society is increasing even though our technology has advanced.

There is no short cut to better health.

The same truths regarding wellness that existed years ago, still, and always will exist.

Either you are involved in the process or you are not.

–87–

What would you change if you were faced with a crisis situation regarding your health?

Why are you waiting?

–88–

Genetically, each one of us is linked to the possibilities of wellness or disease.

Within each of our family trees, there is someone who has had cancer, heart disease, diabetes, or arthritis.

Avoid using their lifestyle as an example for your health.

Stress is the way you respond to internal and external factors in your life.

Stress that causes anxiety, and fear in one person, can cause excitement and enthusiasm in another.

90–

No one makes you sick or gets you upset.

No one can give you a headache.

Your reactions express how your mindbody is responding and functioning.

If you want to improve your health, observe how your emotions respond and how you react to them.

Which serve you and which don't?

–91–

There is no such thing as "just stress."

Your response to stress either weakens your mindbody's neuro-immune system or strengthens it.

–92–

Become familiar with your body.
Know how areas of your body should feel
to touch.

Know where different parts of your body
are on the inside.

It is better for you to discover your body's
discomfort before it discovers you.

–93–

Instead of thinking, "I have a headache or stomachache," say "I hurt in this area."

Ask yourself what have I been thinking, feeling, doing, and eating, or not doing in regards to your health.

–94–

Most health problems do not begin as you get older. They are problems that have been accumulating since childhood.

If you have any dysfunction when you are young, it will have no choice but to continue to get worse as you age if you are not correcting the cause of the problem.

–95–

It does not matter what age you are to begin changing patterns of your lifestyle to improve your health.

Whatever age you are is the time to begin discovering how you can function at a higher level of wellness.

–96–

PREVENTION:

The term, prevention, has been overused in many health care systems today. As the focus remains on preventing illness, we continue to emphasize the problem rather than the solution.

We can have a paradigm shift and focus on wellness creating a greater opportunity of physical, emotional and spiritual health.

WELLNESS FORMULA:

1. Improving the way you think and feel, and how you express your thoughts.
2. Improving the way you eat by understanding proper nutrition.
3. Improving the way you exercise.
4. Improving the way you rest and sleep.
5. Improving the time you spend in prayer and meditation.
6. Seeing a wellness doctor.
7. Taking wellness classes to learn more about physical, emotional, and spiritual healing.
8. Evaluating how well you are following the wellness formula and changing your lifestyle for the better.

Graph your wellness formula

Overall lifestyle _____

Wellness doctor _____

Meditation _____

Rest _____

Exercise _____

Nutrition _____

Self expression _____

Evaluate your consistency as your health is improving.

–99–

BREAKDOWNS IN WELLNESS

1. Worry, fear, anger… on a continued basis, all contribute to the breakdown of wellness.
2. The wrong foods will wear down your mindbody and accumulate toxins in your body.
3. If you are not using a wellness doctor, you are waiting for a crisis.
4. If you are not exercising properly and consistently, you are losing flexibility and strength.
5. If you are not meditating, you are not staying in balance with your higher spirit and wisdom and knowing your connection with God.

–100–

Anytime there is a health problem in your life, or you are feeling fatigued or stressed, you will find at least one of these factors, if not all, out of balance. Begin applying your wellness formula and you will find your health begin to improve.

–101–

Your wellness is top priority. The more you take care of your health, the more your health will take care of you.

With your optimum health, there is nothing you cannot accomplish.

–102–

Specific foods are designed for your mindbody just as specific fuel is meant for your car. Foods will either add to your wellness or to your illness.

–103–

Proper nutrition is good for you whether you are healthy or manifesting illness, or trying to lose weight. The purpose of food is not to fill your appetite but to give your mindbody the potential vitamins, minerals, and energy that enhances your mindbody's optimum performance.

104

Begin to eliminate these foods:

1. Fried foods
2. Bacon, ham, sausage, pork
3. Sandwich meats (processed)
4. Red meat
5. Fast food
6. Soft Drinks
7. White flour products
8. Synthetic foods
9. Foods with artificial coloring, flavoring, preservatives
10. Refined sugar and salt
11. Hot dogs
12. Margarine

Begin to increase these foods:

1. Fruits
2. Vegetables
3. Whole grain foods
4. Legumes
5. If you eat meat then, chicken, turkey, or fish
6. Natural soy products
7. Olive oil
8. Avocados
9. Pure water

Introduce fruit to the morning meal and for snacks, and introduce more vegetables into your lunch and dinner meals. Think like an artist and bring color to your meals. All fruit and vegetables contain specific nutrients to help prevent disease.

Begin to eat organic food

–106–

Become a knowledgeable consumer by reading the ingredients of each food item you purchase.

Do not be fooled by the large print on the packages of food.

–107–

Parents who understand proper nutrition will have an easy time educating their children about healthy foods and its importance.

–108–

When you change your eating habits, have a plan, and specific goals that you and your wellness doctor are committed to.

Natural healing always takes time to obtain the desired results. Learn to enjoy the process of wellness.

–109–

Learn to take the time to bless your food before eating.

Digestion can occur more effectively when you are relaxed with a proper attitude.

–110–

Buy two or three vegetarian cookbooks so that you can see the many various meals you can have without eating meat.

Dine at vegetarian restaurants and begin learning about different foods and preparations.

Ask questions about the different meals, and how they are prepared.

–111–

Do not take supplements as a replacement for healthy nutrition. Supplements are an addition to proper eating.

Your body first wants to receive the proper vitamins and minerals through the digestive process of your food.

–112–

If there is stress to the nervous system, the process of healthy digestion will be interfered with.

Even the best foods will not be digested properly.

–113–

If foods stay in your digestive tract too long, toxins are produced that infiltrate into other parts of the body affecting your health. Most sinus and allergy problems originate from the dysfunction of digestion.

If foods pass too quickly through your digestive tract, you lose the ability to absorb the vital vitamins and minerals that are essential to your health.

EATING GUIDELINES

1. Eat slowly.
2. Drink pure water with fresh lemon daily.
3. Increase raw fruits and vegetables.
4. Do not eat before going to bed.
5. Eat smaller meals more often than eating larger meals.
6. Do not eat when angry or upset.
7. Bring fruit with you to work.
8. Enjoy preparing and eating your food.

–115–

Exercise for at least five minutes every day.

As exercise becomes a part of your lifestyle you will enjoy it more, and plan more time to do it.

Never cause pain while exercising.

Learn to breathe properly while you are stretching, or doing aerobics.

Breathe in slowly and deeply, and exhale slowly while exercising.

If you use weights, use light weights with emphasis on more repetitions.

–117–

When you come home from work, go for a walk and observe nature. This simple exercise revitalizes your energy level, even if your day has seemed stressful.

Allow yourself to feel the bigness of life. The sky, clouds, stars, trees, flowers, and yourself are all a part of this natural world.

–118–

Remember, it is not the stress outside of you that makes you sick, it is the way you internally respond to the stress that makes all the differences in the world.

–119–

Through meditation, you learn how to relax, which is what quiets and disciplines your mindbody. Truly feel the mind and body, your thoughts and feelings as one; functioning together.

Imagine the sound of a finely tuned musical instrument with all the notes in harmony. Imagine your mindbody functioning in harmony.

BREATHING FORMULA:

The more you breathe in,
The more life you draw into your body,
The more you breathe out,
The more toxins you release from your body.

The less you breathe in,
The less life you draw in.
The less you breathe out,
The more toxins you hold inside.

Always begin breathing exercises on your exhalation, breathing everything out, like letting the air out of a balloon, then breathe in slowly.

–121–

When you learn to breathe properly muscles relax, the digestive system assimilates food better, your circulation and heart function easier, your nervous system eases tension, while your energy level increases.

The effect of proper breathing is feeling more connected to yourself, more sensitive to your surroundings, more focused, more creative, and more alive.

–122–

Fear, anger, worry, and anxiety inhabit your breathing, inducing further stress to your mindbody…tightening muscles restricting circulation and pinching nerves, causing you to become more susceptible to injury and sickness.

Take the time to breathe easily and effortlessly.

–123–

Before going to sleep, sit in a meditative posture and listen to your inner voice. Breathe easily and relax, allowing yourself to hear the silence. That inner voice can act as a guide through the many obstacles in life.

Whether you believe in God or a higher power, feel the light of the peacefulness within yourself.

Prayer is speaking to God and meditation is listening to God speaking to you.

–124–

While meditating, learn to release self judgment, self pity, criticism, anger, sadness, and fears, and feel God's unconditional love for you.

This love is not based on what you do, but simply on who you are.

Then allow your own unconditional love for yourself to fill your spirit.

–125–

As your meditations become a lifestyle, develop a forgiving heart.

Healing power is generated through forgiveness. Forgive yourself of all shame, hurt and wrongdoings. When the time is right, forgive others who have hurt you.

−126−

Imagine what you would feel like, and how energetic you would be if you carried no emotional burdens or physical pains, no guilt, no "shoulds," no headaches, or ulcers, no anxiety, no fear of being wrong, or doing wrong.

Imagine feeling good about yourself, not being afraid to express your emotions, and living, giving and sharing your inner love.

Imagine being able to do everything at eighty years old, that you did at eighteen.

… "A Life of Wellness" throughout your life.

BEGINNING AGAIN

It was his time to make the transition soon. His life was filled with wonderful stories, magic, and miracles. Throughout his meanderings of life, the voices guided him when things appeared troubled and dark, as well as through times of joy and love. Each day he talked to the Creator and felt the Creator's presence throughout his being.

As he looked back into the shadow of his life, he saw that there wasn't anything he wished he had done or had not done. His body and mind were still active and healthy, yet he was ready for the passing.

Like a candle's flame that had kept its consistent brightness and pulsing rhythms, he let his body and spirit separate, gently and peacefully, always knowing his home was with the creator.

ABOUT THE AUTHOR

Dr. Marty Finkelstein has been a holistic chiropractor since 1980 specializing in physical, emotional, and spiritual healing and wellness. He has hosted and produced "To Your Health", a cable television show, and hosted "Wake Up To Your Health", an Atlanta radio show. He has been the chiropractic representative for Flying Doctors of America where he teamed with medical doctors, dentists, and other health care professionals providing services to thousands of people in Mexico, Peru, and the Dominican Republic.

Dr. Marty is also the author of:

If Relationships Were Like Sports, Men would at least Know the Score

8 Lessons for Life on Hole 1

Moments in Time- a CD of 15 original songs

Dr. Marty Finkelstein has an office in Decatur, Georgia

To order additional copies of
"A Life of Wellness"

write to:

Dr. Marty Finkelstein
4292-D Memorial Drive
Decatur, Georgia 30032

Or call or e-mail 404-292-6786

drmarty3@yahoo.com

Dr. Marty Finkelstein is available for speaking
engagements and wellness and healing workshops.

LaVergne, TN USA
09 October 2009
160409LV00001BA/6/P